The Kid Who

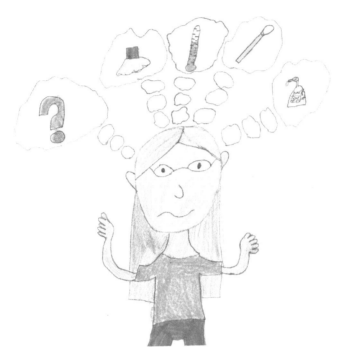

COVID

Authored and Illustrated by Eden Hummel

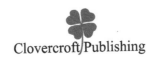

Clovercroft Publishing

Published by Carpenter's Son Publishing, Franklin, Tennessee

Published in association with Larry Carpenter of Christian Book Services, LLC
www.christianbookservices.com

Scripture quotations marked (ESV) are from the ESV® Bible (The Holy Bible, English Standard Version®), copyright © 2001 by Crossway, a publishing ministry of Good News Publishers. Used by permission. All rights reserved.

Edited by Patti Hummel

Cover and Interior Layout Design by Suzanne Lawing

Printed in the United States of America

978-1-950892-99-0

Endorsements

Charming and authentic, this story provides the unique and personal perspective of a young lady who exhibits wisdom beyond her years. Eden informs and encourages in a gentle and humble way, by her example of bravery and her quiet confidence in a time of confusion and uncertainty. As she shares her experience, Eden becomes a model of faith and courage for her peers and for anyone who reads this book. I intend to use it as a platform from which to address the concerns and fears of my own young children.

~**Dr. Clint Archer**, Senior Pastor at Christ Fellowship Baptist Church, Mobile, AL Author, husband, and father to four.

This book is a gem! I've spent 25 years in children's ministry in every possible capacity. Children come is all sorts of sizes and shapes, but they are all vulnerable to fear, especially when that is predominantly what they are hearing. This book breaks through the fear and focuses on Jesus, the Great Physician. This will be a tremendous encouragement to children, as well as parents, who have been touched by the ravages of Covid-19.

~**Diane Leggewie**, Burbank, California, Parent, teacher, author, editor, interim Children's Ministry director, artist.

During this season of unpredictability, grief, and loss, Eden reminds us that no matter what we face we can trust the goodness of God and the love of our family to bring comfort and hope. This honest account of Eden's experience with the COVID-19 virus will help other children and parents as they process the isolation and emotions that comes with a positive test. I'm thankful for the sincere way she expresses her faith in God, and encourages us to do the same.

~**Jason Miller**, Pastor for Children and Families at Grace Community Church, Brentwood, TN, and father of five

Learning how to live through an illness is more important than treatment. That is especially true when there is no universally accepted treatment, but the faith of a child is often more literal than figurative. This is projected in a sweet and, in depth, way in a narrative that tells a brief little account of actions and feelings strongly blended with praye,r and faith, nothing doubting. *The Kid Who Had Covid* is a textbook of faith for the sick child but perhaps for adults to cure experiential doubts also. Thank you, Eden.

~**Jim Carpenter, MD,** Jacksonville, FL.

New words that Eden needed to know and understand the meaning of:

~**Virus**: A virus is a tiny parasite that can only be seen under a microscope. A virus can infect living people and cause disease. It can make copies of itself and spread to humans when they sneeze or breathe on another person.

~**Pandemic**: A disease caused by a virus that can take over the whole country or the world. Often, many people get the disease and many die.

~**COVID-19 Coronavirus**: An illness caused by a virus that can spread from person to person.

~**Virtual School**: An alternative to homeschool that grants students and their parents work with certified teachers and professionally developed online school lessons.

~**Long stick cotton swab**: A cotton swab with a long stick that the doctors use to collect mucus from a person's nose to test for the virus.

~**Protective Mask**: Face masks help prevent the spread of the coronavirus that causes COVID-19. They keep sneezing and coughing germs from spreading through the air.

~**COVID-19 Test Result**: If a COVID-19 test is positive and you do have the virus and you must do what your doctor prescribes. You will need to quarantine.

~**Quarantine**: When a person test positive for the virus they need to be Quarantined. They will stay at home and away from other people who don't have the virus. Quarantine separates and restricts the movement of people who test positive for the virus.

Introduction

The COVID-19 Pandemic of 2020 has impacted the whole world. Many lives have been lost and many of those dear ones died alone. The news has been dismal and confusing to most adults so it's no wonder that children are uncertain and afraid. Children have heard about the Pandemic at school, in their neighborhoods, in their churches, and they have faced changes that alter the way they live their lives. Death is difficult for children, but when they hear about the numbers of people dying from the virus then it hits home, they are not only confused, but afraid.

Eden's dad contracted the virus and was treated while their whole family was quarantined. She learned much during her dad's quarantine that helped to prepare her for some of what she would experience when she contracted the virus a few weeks later at eight years old. She did get afraid, she did feel sadness, and she was lonely. Any one of these emotions would be hard for an eight year old to face.

However, the good thing is that Eden had people in her life to explain the virus to her and to guide her to the source of hope, comfort, and peace. She knew that she could trust Jesus to never leave her, to provide for her, to heal her, and to keep her safe. She wrote this book and drew the illustrations. None of it is perfect, but the hope is, that in her simple way of sharing, others will know Jesus and trust Him to keep them safe and to heal them. God does not allow these things in our lives without purpose, and He will not waste these times, the deep lessons about fear and trust in the midst of the fiery trials. The majority of our trials are not just for us, but for those Jesus leads to us to help in their times of deep trial. Eden's experiences will not be chaff, but wheat to the soul of others. God be glorified!

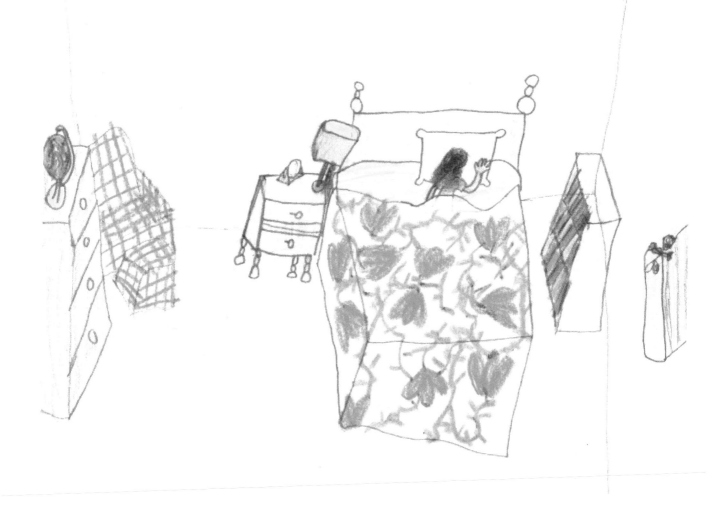

"Mommy, I don't feel well!" I thought I had a little cold. Mommy checked me and I felt hot. I had a stuffy runny nose, and a sore throat. My dad had caught COVID-19 a couple of weeks before, and my family was in quarantine. I told my mommy I wasn't feeling well, and she said maybe it's just a cold, so I went to bed. But mommy wondered...

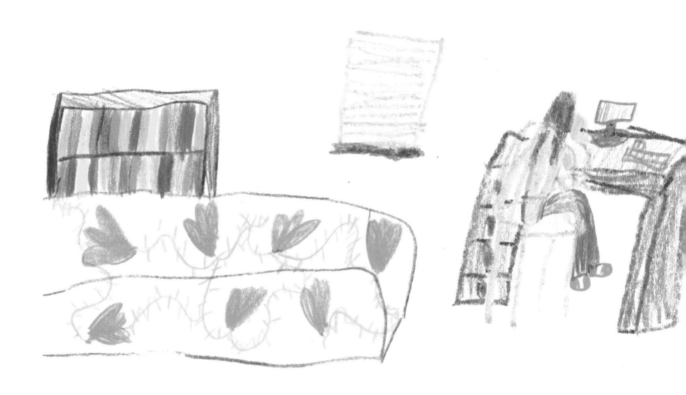

The next day when I got up, I had virtual school. That's when I went on a computer and saw my teacher and did my classwork online. It was a Friday, and I felt even worse! That day, I went through a whole box of tissue! My nose wouldn't stop running! I had a horrible headache. My mom tried to use a thermometer, but it was one of those new digital touchless ones, and she wasn't sure if it worked correctly. We went in the car and drove to the doctor's, so I could get tested for COVID-19.

When we got to the doctor's office, I felt so tired. My mommy and I went back to the exam room. The nurse was very nice, and so was the doctor. The doctor put a long stem cotton swab in my nose and wiggled it around. It tickled a little. The doctor said he would call us when they got the results. I also had to wear a mask to help prevent me from spreading or getting the virus.

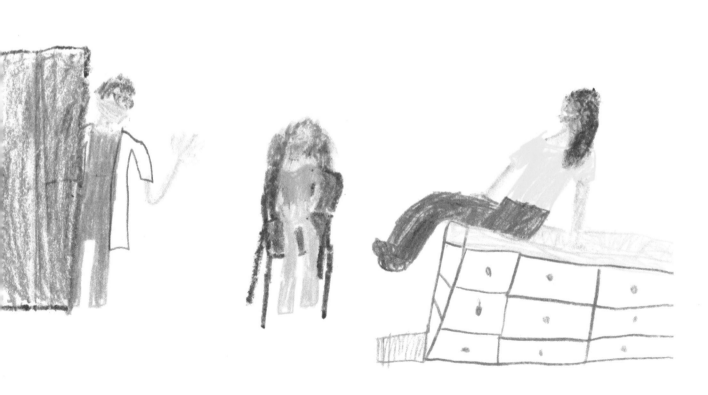

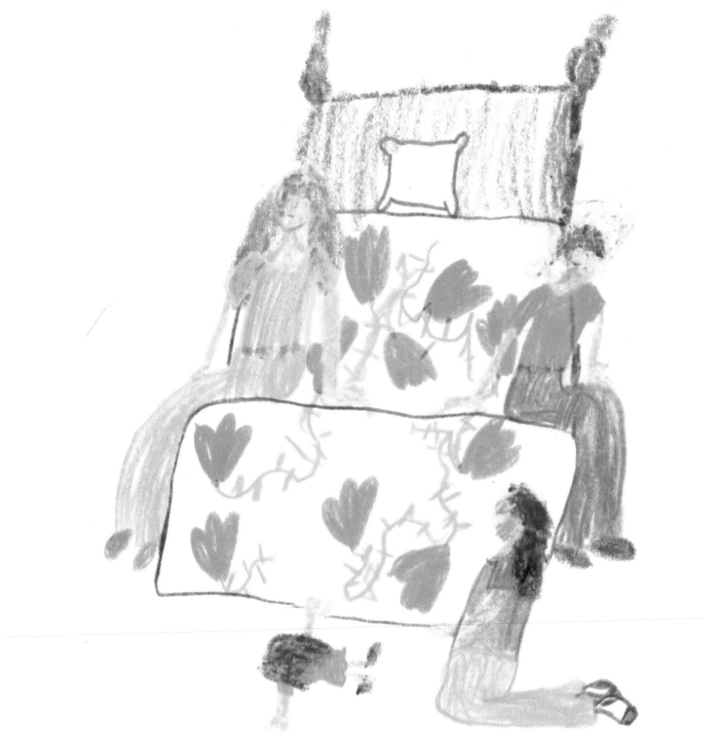

Saturday morning when I woke up and started playing with my dolls in my bedroom, my mommy and dad came in and sat down. I asked them what was going on. They said they got the test results back, and I had COVID-19! I never thought it would happen to us again! First my dad, then me! I was shocked!

That day, my dad set up a television in my room so I could watch movies. I had to stay in my room, away from my brother and my two younger sisters, so hopefully they would not catch the virus, too. My mommy even let me eat French toast in my bedroom! My favorite! But the food tasted weird when I was sick.

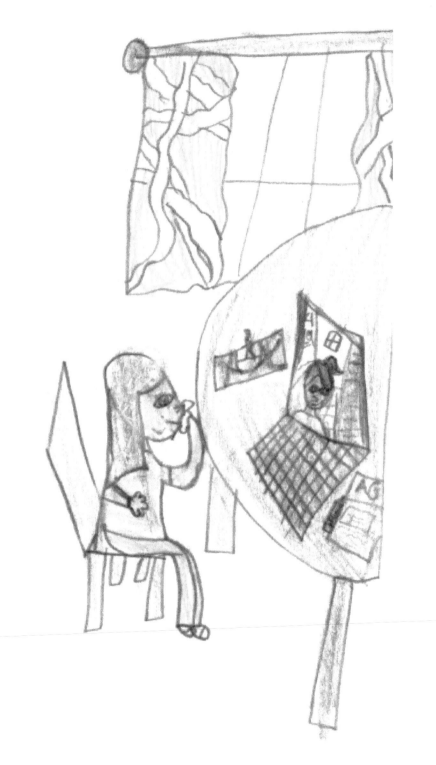

I liked playing with my dolls and watching television while I had to be in my room, but it was lonely. Not playing with my little sisters, Karis and Quinne, or my older brother, Finnley, was boring, and I was kind of sad. I prayed to Jesus every day to please heal me. My grandmother prayed with me over the phone. She told everyone she knew to pray for me. My other grandparents in Florida prayed for me, too. I felt safe because people prayed for me.

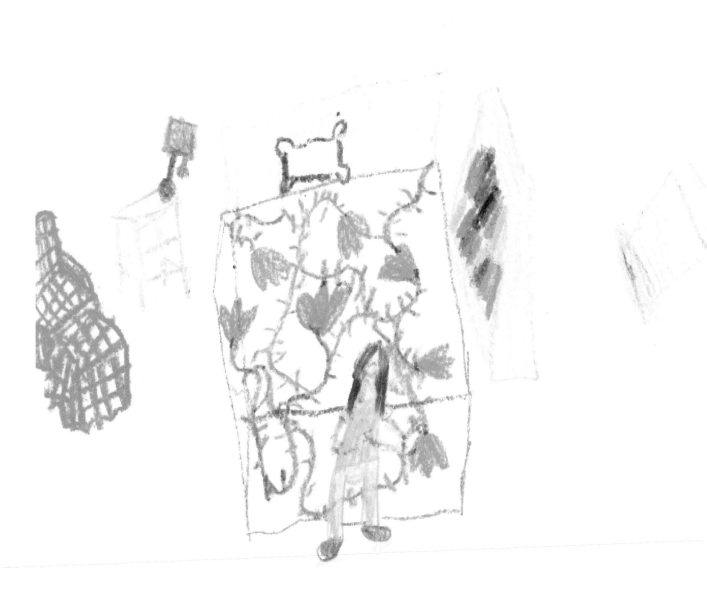

I had COVID-19 all the next week. My mommy kept cleaning and disinfecting everything in the house. It was a lot of work! Thankfully, I eventually felt better, and no one else in my family caught it. When I first learned I had COVID-19 I felt lonely and trapped. But knowing how everyone prayed so much just for me made me realize I will never be alone in this world. And neither will you.

"...fear not, for I am with you; be not dismayed, for I am your God; I will strengthen you, I will help you, I will uphold you with my righteous right hand."

Isaiah 41:10 ESV

"...do not be anxious about anything, but in everything by prayer and supplication with thanksgiving let your requests be made known to God."

Philippians 4-6 ESV

CPSIA information can be obtained
at www.ICGtesting.com
Printed in the USA
JSHW022138300121
11372JS00001B/2

9 781950 892990